穴位按摩治疗高血压

Lowering High Blood Pressure with Acupressure

Normalising your blood pressure in 30 minutes

naturally without prescription drugs

© Charles Chan 2016

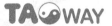

Taoway Publishing - www.taoway.co.uk

1st Edition April 2017

ISBN 978-0-9957419-4-2

Copyright Notice

Disclaimer

This book is intentionally for educational and informational purposes only. The author does not suggest readers self-medicate, self-heal or self-diagnose your medical conditions without consulting a qualified medical practitioner.

Contents

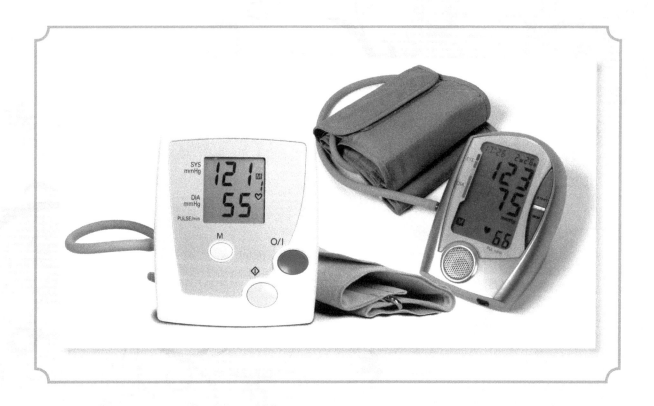

Why is maintaining normal blood pressure important?

Your blood pressure reflects the wellness of your cardiovascular system. If you suffer from hypertension, commonly known as high blood pressure, your heart and blood vessels are subjected to the extra strain and may lead to becoming weaker or damaged. Long-term suffering from high blood pressure without treatment can have serious consequence to your health and may lead to more serious life-threatening conditions:

- It can cause heart attack and heart failure.
- It can cause a stroke or dementia.
- It can cause kidney disease.
- It can cause damage to your eyes.

Understanding your blood pressure

Measuring your blood pressure is very easy nowadays as digital blood pressure devices are very cheap and easily accessible from pharmacists or online stores. When you measure your blood pressure, you will need to pay attention to two results:

1. **Systolic Pressure** (the bigger number) indicates the pressure when your heart pumps blood out.

2. **Diastolic Pressure** (the smaller number) indicates the pressure when your heart is at rest.

Your normal blood pressure should be between 90/60 and 140/90 during the period when you are not physically active. Generally speaking, the younger you are, the lower your blood pressure you should have. Blood pressure can fluctuate and have big variations with the reading throughout the whole day as it reflects how hard your heart is working and what you have consumed. For example, your blood pressure will go up if you have been exercising or under stress and it will go down if you are calm or at rest. Generally speaking, your blood pressure is at the lowest during sleep when your body is inactive, and it will increase when you are awakened and become active. Your blood pressure can also be affected by consuming salt, fatty food, caffeine or alcohol. It can also be affected if you have not been drinking enough. Therefore, it is important to measure your blood pressure only when you are calm and restful, and you are not dehydrated or over-consuming salt, caffeine, fatty food or alcohol. To get a more accurate blood pressure reading, you should measure your blood pressure at least three times with a couple of minutes gap between taking each reading. You should never take the first reading as the final score. If the reading remains higher than the normal score, you should do the acupressure treatment to normalise the pressure.

About Acupressure

Acupressure is an ancient Chinese healing art derives from acupuncture which was developed over 5000 years ago. Similar to acupuncture using needles on the vital energy points of the meridians, acupressure uses only the fingers to massage on the energy points which activates the body to relieve the symptoms and to heal itself. Acupressure massage is very effective in lowering blood pressure, increasing circulation and vitality, relieving pains and aches, reducing stress and is a superb self-treatment for boosting the body immunity and it is a safe alternative self-healing modality.

About the Acupressure massage routine

These massage exercises have been widely practised in China because they are renown for the effectiveness and positive instantaneous results. They are very easy to learn. You can perform your treatment at your own leisure in your own environment, and you do not require any props to aid your treatment.

There are altogether nine exercises. Apart from Exercise 1, you can perform these exercises with any sequence of your preference. All you need is to perform these exercises once a day but if you have time you could certainly do it more than once a day. The full set of routine will take roughly twenty to thirty minutes. The result is instantaneous. You can certainly increase the duration by increasing the repetitions of the routine. You can also monitor your own progress by measuring your blood pressure before and after performing the routine. In most cases, the systolic pressure will become normalised or have a significant drop after performing a basic twenty to a thirty-minute routine. Diastolic pressure will also have a significant drop corresponding to the systolic pressure drop.

Exercise 1 - 调息 Regulation of breath

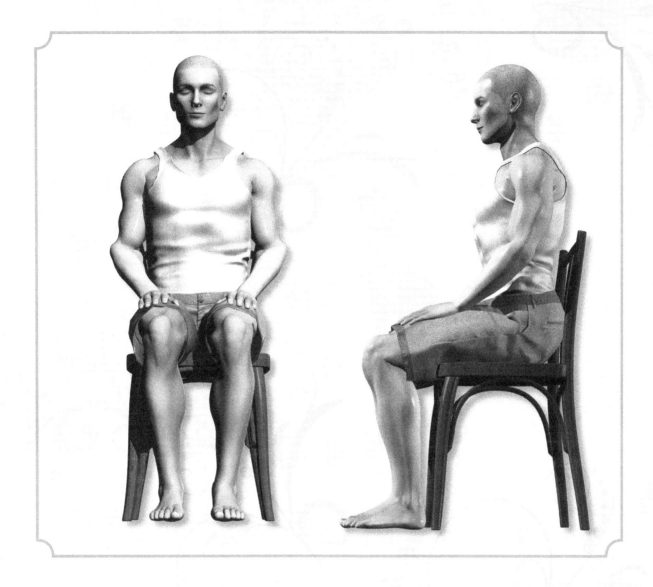

This is a breathing exercise to be performed before and after each massage routine. Use your diaphragm to breathe. Breathe in with your nostrils and breathe out with your mouth.

1.   Sit on a chair and keep your body straight. Put your hands on your laps and keep your shoulders relaxed.

2.   Close your eyes and allow your facial muscles to relax into a happy smile. You can induce your smile by thinking of a memorable happy event, such as a special childhood birthday party, a reunion Christmas gathering or a graduation event.

3.   Breathe gently, slowly, and naturally, but prolong and deepen your breaths using diaphragmatic movements. Don't force anything unnatural. Deep diaphragmatic breathing occurs automatically once your body is totally relaxed. The more you are relaxed, the deeper your breathing will become. If you are doing this exercise correctly, your belly will balloon up naturally when inhaling and it will flatten when exhaling. While you are doing the diaphragmatic breathing, observe your thoracic movement. Pay attention to your chest, and your rib cage should have minimal movement while all the motions should happen on your belly.

4.   Perform this breathing exercise for two to three minutes. You can certainly do it longer. It is a very enjoyable experience as it puts your mind into a meditative consciousness.

Exercise 2 - Massage 百会 Pai Hui point

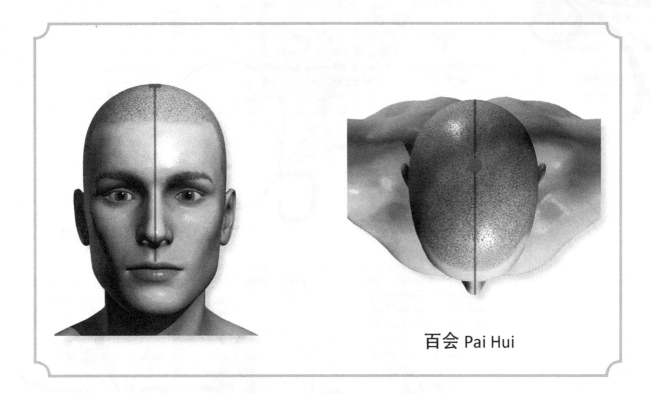

百会 Pai Hui

百会 **Pai Hui** point is the centre point on top of your skull. It is located on the 督脉 **Governing Meridian** which runs from the middle of the top lip towards the middle bottom of the perineum area. **Pai Hui** means **Hundred Gatherings**; it is a very important point for lowering the excessive **Yang** energy which often referring to be an excessive fire in the liver. The excessive fire in the liver is the Chinese terminology equivalent to hypertension in Western medical terminology. Therefore to massage, the **Pai Hui** point can bring about lowering the blood pressure by balancing the **Yang Qi** (Chi).

1.   Put both hands on top of your head and use the fingertips of the index, middle and ring fingers to massage the point in circular motions gently.

2.   Breathe gently, calmly and naturally with the diaphragmatic movements.

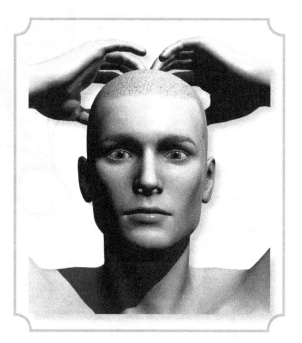

3.   Massage this area for two to three minutes.

4.   Then put your palms on the laps and repeat the breathing exercise of **Exercise 1** for a minute or two.

Exercise 3 - Massage front and back of the skull

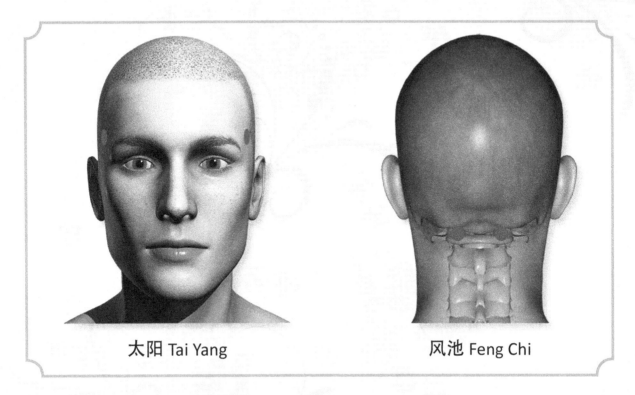

太阳 Tai Yang   风池 Feng Chi

For this exercise, you will massage the forehead front, temple areas and also the occipital area covering the 太阳 **Tai Yang** points on temple area on both sides of your head and 风池 **Feng Chi points** at the bottom of the skull on the occipital area. **Tai Yang** points are very effective in treating facial paralysis, temporal headache and migraine headache. The **Feng Chi** points rest on the left and right 胆经 **Gall Bladder Meridians** on the occipital area between the lower part of your skull and neck. These points are very effective for treating occipital headache, paralysis, stress-related tension on the shoulder areas.

1.   Rub both palms together until they become hot.

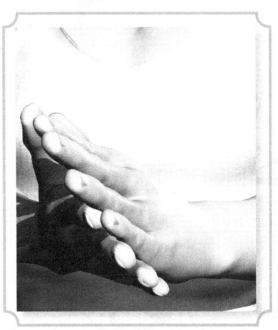

2.   Now rest the muscular area below your thumbs of your palms (**Thenar Eminence**) in the middle of your forehead.

3.   Gently, smoothly and simultaneously move them backwards, rubbing the temple areas, and with your thumbs moving back on the top of your ears.

4.   Now follow the rim of the bottom of your skull until your thumbs sink into the indentation areas. Rest all other fingers on the occipital area of the skull on the back of your head. The indentation areas are the 风池 **Feng Chi** points.

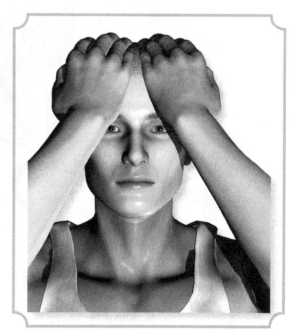

5.   Then use the thumbs to massage the indentation areas in circular motions for ten to thirty times.

6.   Repeat steps 2 to 4.

7.   Then put your palms on the laps and repeat the breathing exercise of **Exercise 1** for a minute or two.

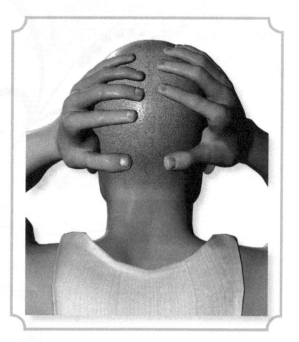

Exercise 4 - Massage 人迎 Ren Ying points

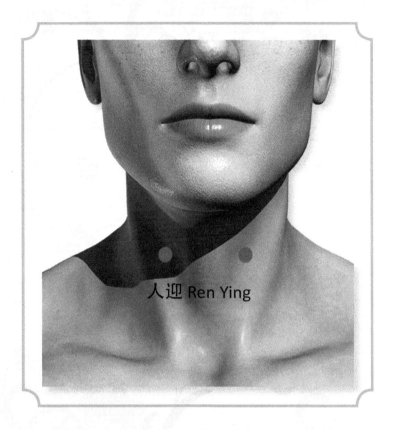

人迎 Ren Ying

人迎 **Ren Ying points** are located on both sides of the neck where the pulse of the carotid artery can be felt. **Ren Ying** points rest on the left and right 胃经 **Stomach Meridians,** and they are very effective for calming the blood pressure as well as treating headache and dizziness as a result of the imbalance of the **Liver Qi** (Chi).

1. Rub both palms together especially concentrate on the index, middle and ring finger areas until they become hot.

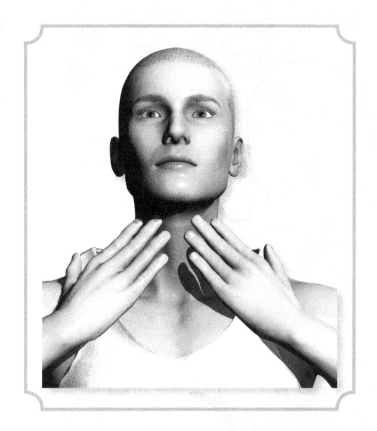

2.   Place the three fingers of both hands on the **Ren Ying** area where you can feel the pulses.

3.   You can close your eyes while doing this exercise. Massage gently with circular motions either clockwise or anti-clockwise for at least thirty times. You can extend the length of the massage as long as you wish.

4.   If your blood pressure is high, you would feel the pulses are forceful and fast. These points are very effective in calming the blood pressure, and you should be able to feel the forcefulness of the pulses calming down after massaging for a while.

5.   Once again return your palms on your laps and perform the breathing exercise of **Exercise 1** for a minute or two.

Exercise 5 - Massage 膻中 Dan Zhong and 巨阙 Ju Que points

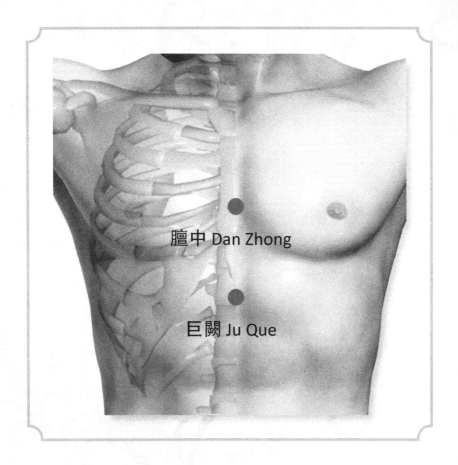

膻中 **Dan Zhong** and 巨阙 **Ju Que** are both located on the 任脉 **Conception Meridian** in the middle front of the body. **Dan Zhong** is located in the middle of the sternum levels with the nipples with men. For women, you can locate it by feeling the groove between the fourth and fifth ribs from the collar bone counting downward. **Dan Zhung** is levelled with the groove in the middle of the sternum.

Ju Que is right below **Dan Zhung**. It is located about an inch (2.5 cm) below the tip of the sternum in the middle of the solar plexus area. Both **Dan Zhung** and **Ju Que** points can bring about calming the spirit and alleviating angina.

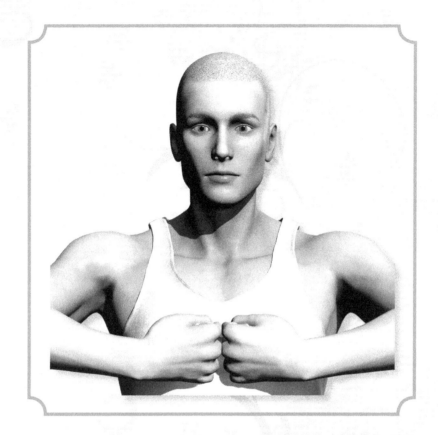

1.   To massage these two points, use the second knuckles of all four fingers while holding a loose fist.

2.   Rub the **sternum** and **Solar Plexus** areas vertically with an up and down movement using middle firm pressure.

3.   You can massage with one fist or both fists together.

4.   You should feel the heat emitting from the massaged area after massaging for two to three minutes.

5.   Put your palms on your laps and perform the breathing exercise of **Exercise 1** for another minute or two.

Exercise 6 - Massage along the 心经 Heart Meridian

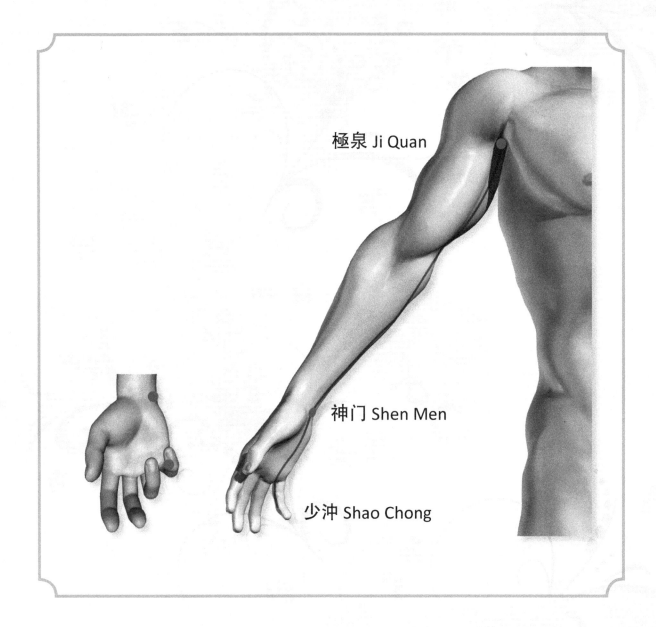

極泉 Ji Quan

神门 Shen Men

少沖 Shao Chong

心经 **Heart Meridian** is located on the inside edge of both arms running from underneath the armpit to the inside edge of the little finger. **Heart Meridian** as the name suggested, it governs the functions of the heart organ as well as the human spirit (mental health) according to the Chinese medical doctrine.

1. Use the right thumb supported by other fingers to massage the left **Heart Meridian**.

2. Apply medium pressure and do small circular motion while pressing downward.

3. Starting from the first point 極泉 **Ji Quan** underneath the armpit and work your way down towards the little finger moving an inch (2.5 cm) a time until you have reached 少沖 **Shao Chong**, the final point on **Heart Meridian** on the tip of the little finger.

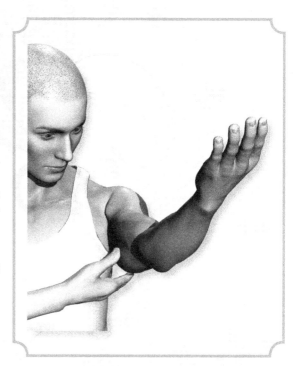

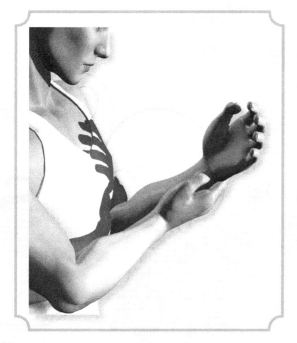

4. Spend a little bit longer and put a bit more emphasis on the wrist line area where 神门 **Shen Men** point is located at the crease of the wrist, about a quarter of an inch (1 cm) inside.

5. **Shen Men** can be translated as the Spirit Door. It is a very important point for calming the spirit as well as having a high impact of normalising blood pressure.

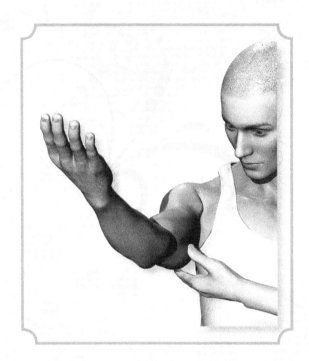

6.   You can run through the massage along the **Heart Meridian** two or three times.

7.   Then repeat the procedures above and massage your right **Heart Meridian** using your left thumb.

8.   Put your palms on your laps and perform the breathing exercise of **Exercise 1** for another minute or two.

Exercise 7 - Massage 合谷 He Gu point

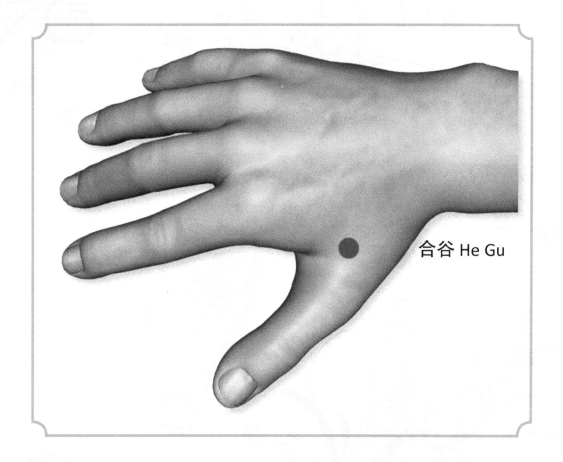

合谷 **He Gu** Point is a very important point on the 大肠经 **Large Intestine Meridian** for clearing the wind, heat, pain, skin eruptions and lowering blood pressure. To locate **He Gu**, when you turn your palm facing downward, it is at the dorsum of the hand between the first and second metacarpal bones, roughly in the middle of the second metacarpal bone on the radial side.

1.   Use your thumb and the index finger to pinch the point with medium to strong pressure and at the same time use the thumb to massage the point with a rotational movement for a minute or so.

2.   You should feel a dull achy sensation on the **He Gu** location. If you cannot tolerate the dull ache, press with less pressure to begin with and build your pressure up gradually.

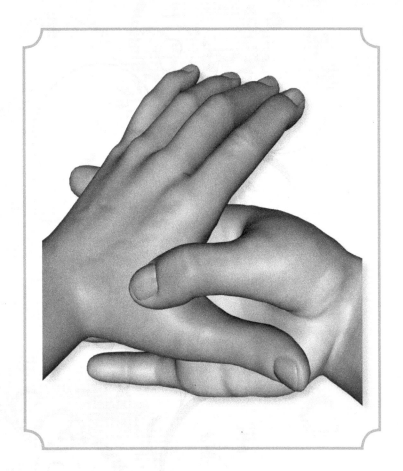

3. Massage the **He Gu** point on both hands.

4. Put your palms on your laps and perform the breathing exercise of **Exercise 1** for another minute or two.

Exercise 8 - Massage 命门 Ming Men point and the kidney regions

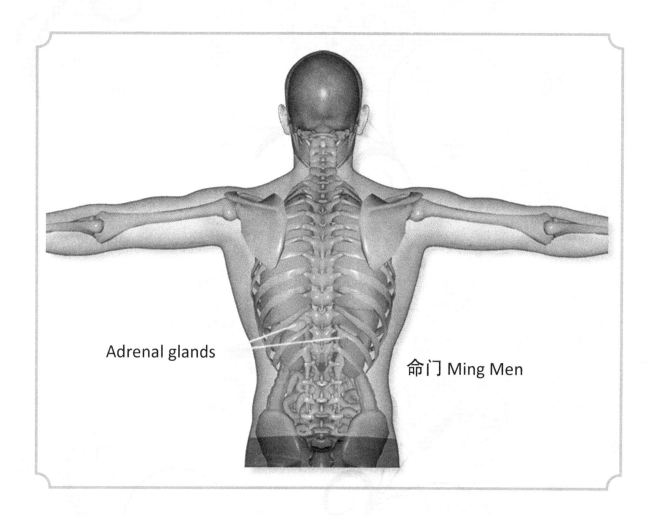

Adrenal glands

命门 Ming Men

The kidneys are located on the two sides of your back roughly at the lower rib area. There is an important point in the middle of the spine called **命门 Ming Men** or **Door of Life** in English. This point is located near the adrenal gland areas which are fundamental to alleviate fatigue and stress and revitalise the **kidney Qi** (Chi). **Kidney Qi** or kidney energy is the primal sexual energy in Chinese medicine which governs the overall vitality and well-being.

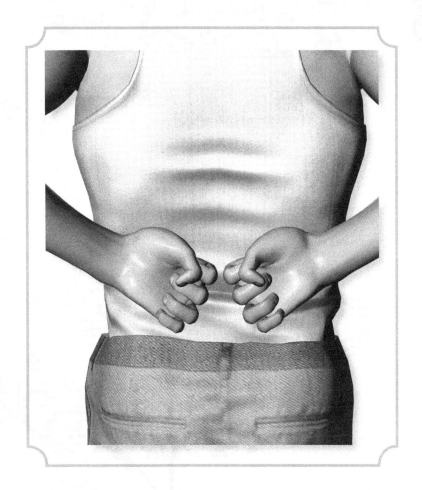

1. Hold both hands into loose fists and use the back of the fists to rub the kidney areas using an up and down movement. Continue the massage for a minute or two.

2. Repeat the breathing exercise of **Exercise 1** by putting your palms on your laps for a minute or two.

Exercise 9 - Massage 足三里 Zu San Li, 三阴交 San Yin Jiao and 涌泉 Young Quan points

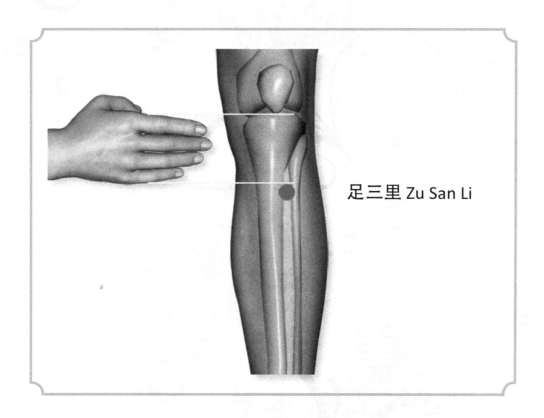

足三里 Zu San Li

足三里 **Zu San Li** is situated on the 胃经 **Stomach Meridian**, at a four finger width distance under the kneecap on the outside edge of your tibia (shin bone). **Zu San Li** is a very important point for lowering hypertension. Massaging this point will nourish **Qi and Blood**. It is also especially effective for treating problems with digestion including diarrhoea, constipation, abdominal pain and other ailments in the gastric-intestinal tract.

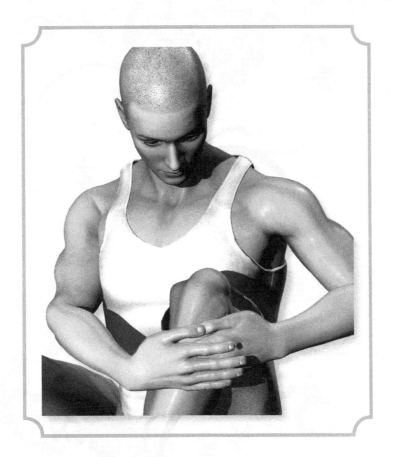

1. Use your thumb and apply deep pressure to massage **Zu San Li** point with a rotational movement.

2. You should feel a dull achy sensation in this location. If you cannot tolerate the dull ache, press with less pressure to begin with and build your pressure up gradually.

3. Once you can tolerate the dull ache, use both hands to apply even deeper pressure. If you use your right-hand thumb to do the massage, you can apply the left-hand thumb on top of the right-hand thumb to increase the pressure. Some people feel easier to use the left-hand index finger and middle finger to assist the right-hand thumb which is also okay, as long as you feel whichever way easier or more natural for you.

4. Massage this point on both legs for one to two minutes and then move down to 三阴交 the **San Yin Jiao** point.

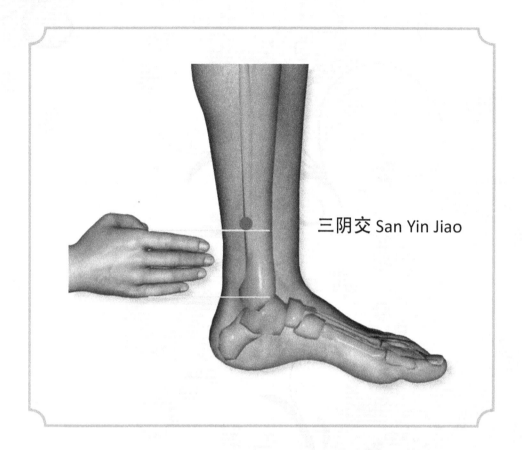

三阴交 **San Yin Jiao** is located on the 脾经 **Spleen Meridian**. It is four finger width distance on the edge of the tibia above the centre of the inside ankle. The major functions of **San Yin Jiao** are to nourish the spleen, cleanse the liver and strengthen the kidneys. Kidneys in Chinese medicine are normally referring to the sexual sphere. Therefore this is an important point for treating digestive disorders related to the spleen, sexual problems for men and women and problems caused by excessive liver energy, such as hypertension, palpitation, insomnia and anxiety.

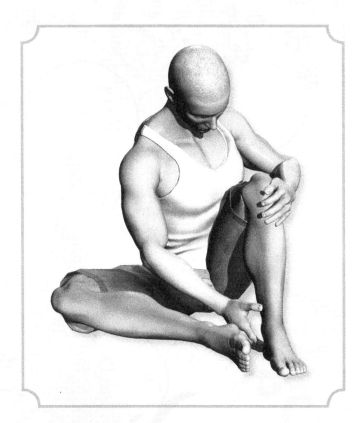

1. Use your thumb and apply deep pressure to massage this point with a rotational movement.

2. You should feel a dull achy sensation on the massaged location. If you cannot tolerate the dull ache, press with less pressure to begin with and build your pressure up gradually.

3. Once you can tolerate the dull ache, use both hands to apply even deeper pressure. If you use your right-hand thumb to do the massage, you can apply the left-hand thumb on top of the right-hand thumb to increase the pressure. Some people feel easier to use the left-hand index finger and middle finger to assist the right-hand thumb which is also okay, as long as you feel whichever way easier or more natural for you.

4. Massage this point on both legs for one to two minutes and then move down to **涌泉 Young Quan** point.

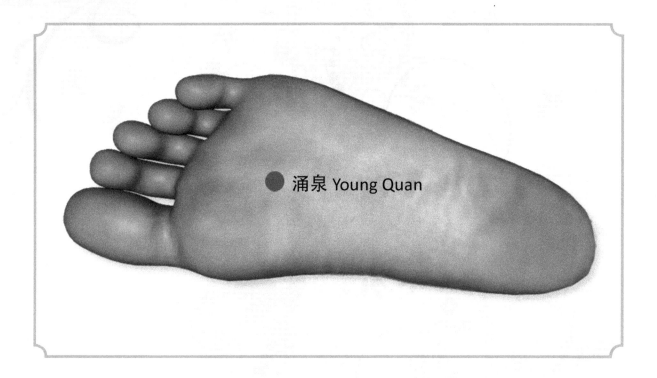

涌泉 Young Quan point is the first point on the **肾经 Kidney Meridian** which is located in the centre of depression between the darker skin of the sole and the paler skin of the arch on the bottom of your feet. Apart from treating hypertension, it is very effective for treating fainting, loss of consciousness, tension on back and neck, asthma, headache and stomach ache.

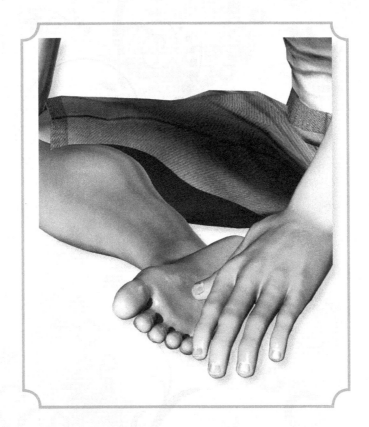

1. Use your thumb and apply deep pressure to massage this point with a rotational movement.

2. You should feel a dull achy sensation on the massaged location. If you cannot tolerate the dull ache, press with less pressure to begin with and build your pressure up gradually.

3. Once you can tolerate the dull ache, use both hands to apply even deeper pressure. If you use your right-hand thumb to do the massage, you can apply the left-hand thumb on top of the right-hand thumb to increase the pressure. Some people feel easier to use the left-hand index finger and middle finger to assist the right-hand thumb which is also okay, as long as you feel whichever way easier or more natural for you.

4. Massage this point on both feet for one to two minutes. Then put your palms on the laps and repeat the breathing exercise of **Exercise 1** for two to five minutes to finish off the whole routine.

Long-term prevention and treatment of hypertension

High blood pressure itself is not an illness. It is caused by physiological, psychological and chemical factors or a combination of these factors. These factors are closely related to your lifestyle. High blood pressure is merely a symptom when your body is telling you something is not right, and you need to listen to your body to make changes so as to stop injuring your body any further. The following are the major factors that may contribute to the elevation of your blood pressure:

- **Your body weight**

- **Diet and lifestyle**

- **Excessive caffeine intake**

- **Excessive alcohol consumption**

- **Insufficient sleep**

- **Long term stress**

- **Diabetes**

- **Medication or oral contraceptives**

- **Cardiovascular health**

Acupressure massage is an excellent way to relax your heart and dilates your blood vessels to alleviate the abnormal blood pressure, but it does not eliminate the root causes if you are doing something continuously to injuring your body. For long term and lasting cure, one needs to take steps to eliminate all the root causes. As you can see from above, many factors can contribute to the elevation of your blood pressure and in many ways they are co-related and must be dealt with simultaneously.

Weight gain and hypertension

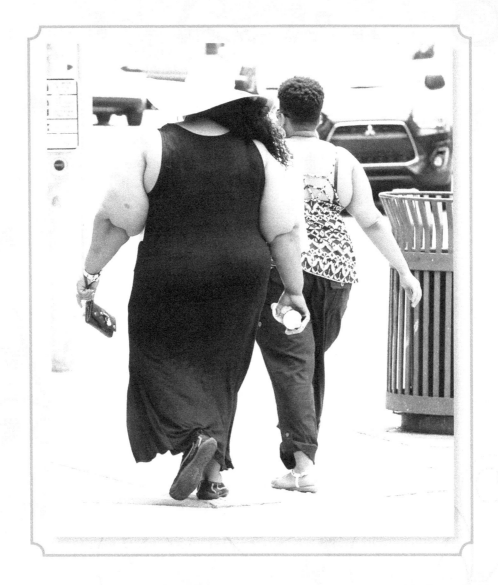

If you are overweight or in the obese category, you are most likely to endanger yourself from a whole host of health issues apart from high blood pressure.

If you are overweight or in the obese category, you are most likely to endanger yourself from a whole host of health issues apart from high blood pressure, including type 2 diabetes, high blood cholesterol, metabolic syndrome, osteoarthritis, breathing disorder, gallstone, reproductive problems, cancers, stroke and coronary heart diseases. As your body mass index rises, so does your risk for developing cardiovascular diseases. A waxy substance called plaque builds up inside your arteries and narrowing your body pipework. Your heart requires working much harder to pump enough blood to your body and as a result of the narrowing of your arteries, your blood pressure elevates. If insufficient blood is pumped to your heart, it can cause angina or heart attack. If plaques rupture, it can cause the formation of blood clots which can block blood flow within your body. In either of these cases, if a clot blocks a blood vessel of the heart, it will cause a heart attack, and if a clot blocks a blood vessel in the brain, it will cause a stroke.

Therefore it is crucial to keep your body trim and your body mass index within the normal range. You can calculate your body mass index with this online BMI calculator:

http://www.nhs.uk/Tools/Pages/Healthyweightcalculator.aspx

A body mass index is considered to be normal if it is between 18.5 and 24.9. You are overweight if your BMI is 25 to 29.9 and you are obese if your BMI is over 30.

Stop comfort eating

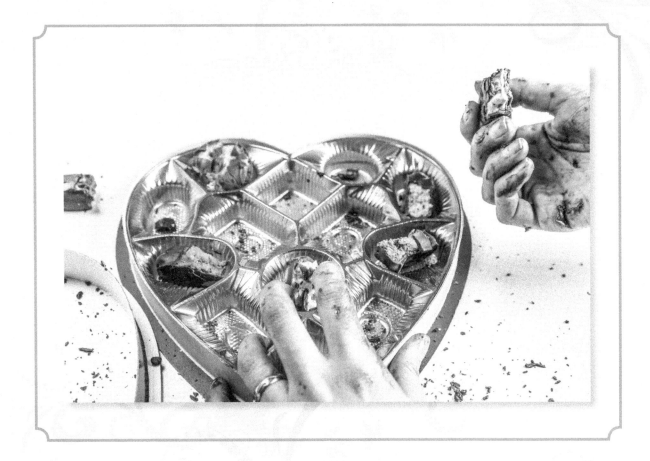

People who are eating excessively or compulsively are suffered from Binge Eating Disorder. People with Binge Eating Disorder may suffer from emotional trauma, low self-esteem or depression. They turn to food for comfort to cover up their underlining unhappiness or unresolved emotional issues.

Binge eating may give the sufferers a brief moment of comfort or a sense of gaining control while they are on the binge, but often the sense of guilt and regret will overwhelm them when the reality sets in. The more the hurt they feel, the more they use food to regain comfort and control. People with binge eating disorder often gain weight leading to a vast number of health issues, such as obesity, high blood pressure, high cholesterol, type 2 diabetes, arthritis, cancer and cardiovascular diseases. It is therefore very important to recognise the root cause of your emotional problem and seek professional help.

Consider changing to a plant-based diet

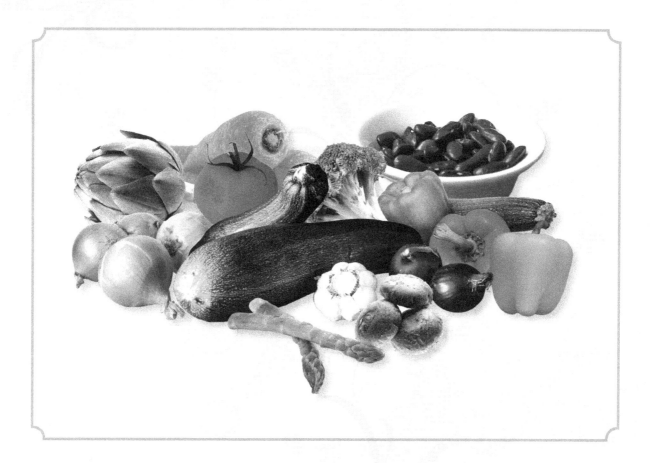

A strong science-based body of evidence indicates plant-based diet promotes good health and longevity and has healing effects on reversing chronic conditions such as cardiovascular diseases, hypertension, diabetes, kidney diseases, arthritis, and even cancers. Seventh Day Adventists who have been vegetarians/vegans for over a century and ban using tobacco and alcohol, live an average of 10 years longer than most Americans and even at an advanced age, they still enjoy good health physically, mentally and spiritually.

Dr T. Colin Campbell[Ref 1] conducted a large-scale study known as the China Study[Ref 2] in 1980 with the help from a Chinese scientist Dr Junshi Chen to explore the relationship between nutrition and chronic conditions such as cancers, heart, and metabolic diseases. They gather data from 6500 people from sixty-five rural and semi-rural counties and found more than 8,000 statistically significant associations between lifestyle, diet, and diseases. All the scientific evidence is pointing towards the benefits of plant-based lifestyle for optimum health and to prevent and reverse diseases such as diabetes, cardiovascular diseases and cancers.

Former President of the USA Bill Clinton underwent emergency heart surgery of implanting two coronary stents in his heart in 2010 after previously underwent a quadruple bypass surgery in 2004. After reading Dr Dean Ornish's Program for Reversing Heart Disease[Ref 3], Dr Caldwell Esselstyn's Prevent and Reverse Heart Disease[Ref 4] and Dr T. Colin Campbell's China Study[Ref 2], Clinton took on a plant-based diet, lost 25 pounds and kept the weight off. After doing some research, he realised that 82% of the people who made a drastic change to their diet, their bodies would heal themselves. Their arterial blockage cleans up, the calcium deposit around their heart breaks up. The arterial blockages and plaques are the major factors of causing hypertension and cardiovascular diseases. By changing your diet, you can eliminate not only high blood pressure but also the cause of many serious diseases.

Are you consuming too much alcohol or caffeine?

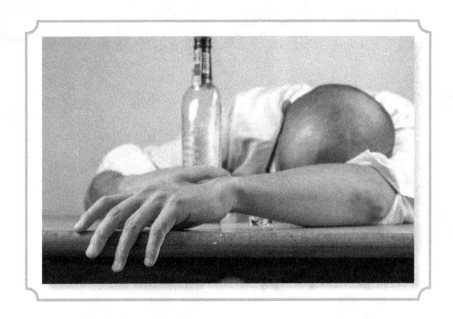

Both alcohol and caffeine have diuretic properties and can cause body dehydration if drunken excessively.

Dehydration can trigger sodium retention, and the body will then close some capillary beds as a result, causing increased blood pressure in the arteries. Drinking too much alcohol can instantly raise your blood pressure to unhealthy levels, especially if you are a binge drinker, your habit could lead to long-term elevation of blood pressure. If you are a heavy drinker who wants to quit or reduce drinking alcohol, you should consider gradually reducing your consumption over one to two weeks because if you stop drinking suddenly it may lead to developing severe high blood pressure for several days.

If you have high blood pressure for stress or other medical reasons, you should avoid alcohol altogether. Drinking alcohol can also lead to heart and liver diseases anyway. Studies have also shown a rise in breast cancer risk in women under 50 from drinking alcohol even light or moderate drinking could have a bearing on developing breast cancer. Therefore, do take note of the recommendations of moderate alcohol consumption below:

- Two drinks a day for men younger than age 50

- One drink a day for men age 50 and older

- One drink or none a day for women of any age

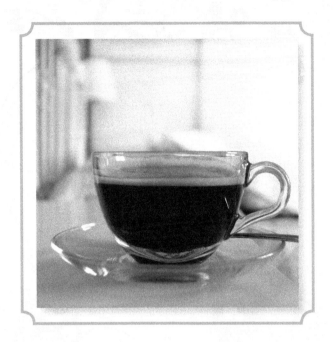

Consuming too much caffeine can cause short-term elevation of blood pressure even if your blood pressure is generally normal.

This may be due to its diuretic properties, or it causes more adrenaline to release leading to heart rate acceleration. This is not a problem if you are generally healthy, but it may be an issue for those with underlying health issues like heart disease, hypertension or Arrhythmia (irregular heartbeat). Too much caffeine may also over-stimulate your central nervous system leading to insomnia. Insufficient sleep is also one of the root causes of hypertension. The lack of sleep can have very detrimental effects on your mental well-being as it may lead to anxiety, mood swings and even depression.

Therefore, avoid consuming caffeine excessively and especially if you have high blood pressure in the first place, consider avoiding any caffeinated beverages, including coffee, tea, or certain soda pops altogether.

Insufficient sleep and hypertension

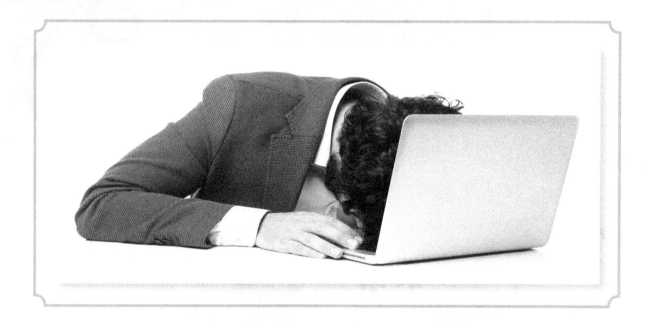

Melatonin is a natural hormone produced by the pineal gland in your brain. During the day the pineal gland is inactive, only traces of melatonin can be detected in your bloodstream. When it becomes dark in the evening, the pineal gland switches on and secretes melatonin actively into the blood. Melatonin secretion happens from around 9 pm to 11 pm every evening. As your melatonin level in the blood rises, you begin to feel sleepy. Your body requires sleep to lowering the blood pressure, replenishing itself, lowering stress and repairing your heart and blood vessels.

Studies show that long-term insufficient sleep can have dramatic health consequences. Insufficient sleep may have a link to weight gain (see **Weight gain and hypertension** on page 33), a greatly increased risk of having or developing type 2 diabetes, an increased risk of cardiovascular diseases including hypertension, stroke, coronary heart diseases, and Arrhythmia (irregular heartbeat).

If you have a problem of insomnia or not able to have a deep sleep, you should look into the causes or make changes to your lifestyle or your daily routine:

- Eat your supper at least 3 hours before you go to bed and avoid having a heavy or greasy meal.

- Avoid having a hot bath or shower before going to bed as they will increase your alertness and keep you awake.

- Avoid drinking strong tea, coffee and caffeinated soda pop during the day and especially near your bedtime.

- Shut the curtains and keep your bedroom dark as darkness stimulates secretion of Melatonin.

- Consider taking Passiflora, Valerian and Magnesium Chloride or Citrate supplements. These supplements help to relax your body, easing your anxiety, lowering your blood pressure and improving the quality of your sleep.

- Open some windows to ensure good ventilation in your bedroom and to keep the atmosphere cool.

- Are there any underlining problems bothering you? Are you worrying about your finance or something else? If you do, recognise that you might be stressed (see next section on stress reduction).

Reduce your stress level

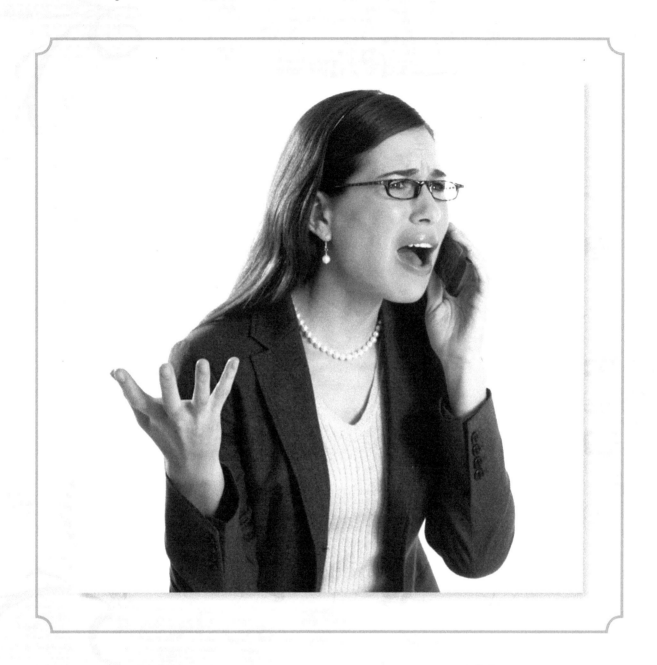

Stress is a combination of emotional, physiological and psychological effects caused by a build-up of pressure, worry or unhappiness.

Stress is a combination of emotional, physiological and psychological effects caused by a build-up of pressure, worry or unhappiness. When you are under pressure, your body will exercise a survival instinct called fight or flight response. This fight or flight response is most invaluable when you are facing life-threatening dangers to your physical survival.

The fight or flight response is an evolutionary survival instinct for the event of an emergency. When you are confronted with a dangerous situation, your hypothalamus in your brain sends out a signal to your adrenal glands, and within seconds of surging the survival hormone adrenaline, you are able to run faster, hit harder, yell louder, hear and see sharper, more than you normally could. Your heart rate pumps at twice the normal speed to release reserved energy to all your major muscles in your arms and legs.

All other major functions of your body such as digestion and reproduction etc. are temporarily shut down in order to give you a better chance of survival. This fight or flight response is most invaluable when we are confronted with a life-threatening danger to our physical survival. Today, most of the dangers we have to confront are not life-threatening situations but our evolutionary instinct is still continuously responding as if they are life-threatening to our survival. Stress can affect your heart, kidneys, digestion, sleep pattern, psychological and mental well-being. Chronic stress can have drastic effects on your health and can be leading to more serious illnesses such as adrenal fatigue, cancers, depression, cardiovascular diseases and hypertension. Therefore, if you have prolonged fears, sadness, feelings of helplessness, uncontrollable anger bursts, tension on your back, shoulders and back, chronic headaches, all these are pointing to you may be suffering from chronic stress. You need to examine your life carefully and find out what are the triggers of your stress.

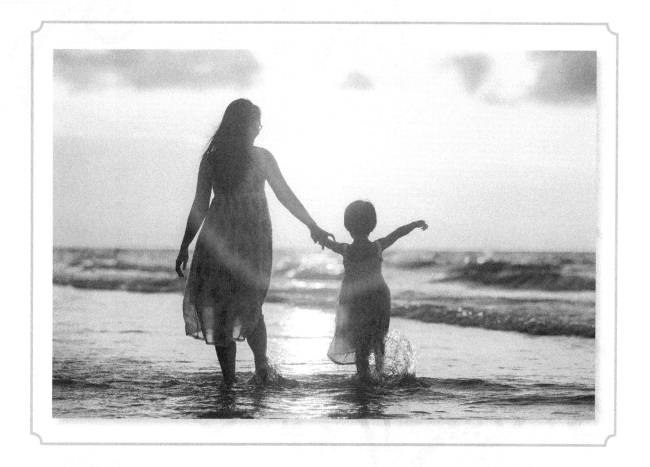

There are things you can do and steps to take to reduce your stress level:

- Practise meditation, Qi Gong or Tai Chi. They are the most effective antidotes for stress as they can bring about the total and holistic health benefits of harmonising your body, mind and spirit.

- Prioritise and organise routines for both home and work. Try to make a happy medium.

- Be organised, and you will save time and avoid creating last-minute anxiety.

- Have fun, take a break or have a change of scenery. Don't just work to make a living but work to enjoy living.

- If you are not happy with your current job, consider a change of career orientation. Don't procrastinate and take action now before you are totally stressed out.

- A good night sleep allows your body to recuperate, to absorb and assimilate nutrition and to regenerate new cells. A bad night sleep is detrimental to your temper, your mental health, your physical health and your concentration at work the following day.

- Exercise relieves stress and produces endorphins; the happy hormones in the brain which make you feel relaxed and happy.

- Reduce consumption of stress-induced stimulants. Caffeine, sugar, alcohol and nicotine are all adrenal stimulants that can trigger a stress response in the body even when no major external stress is present.

- Have a good wholesome plant-based diet. Cut out eating package food and junk food as they are usually, high in salt, sugar, and trans fats that can make you fat and cause inflammation to your circulatory system. They are also packed with artificial additives, such as preservatives to extend shelf life, artificial colourings and flavour enhancers to entice you to have more. These additives may cause allergic respiratory reactions, such as asthma, rhinitis; skin problems, such as rash, hives or itching and digestive disorders, such as diarrhoea and stomach pains. The worse of all, they can cause, mental and behavioural disorders such as hyperactivity, attention deficit hyperactivity disorder (ADHD), insomnia and irritability.

- Learn to slow down your pace of life and understand life is not an emergency.

- Look for help professionally or get social support from your family and friends and don't bottle up your problems and anxiety and pretending you are coping alright.

Diabetes and hypertension

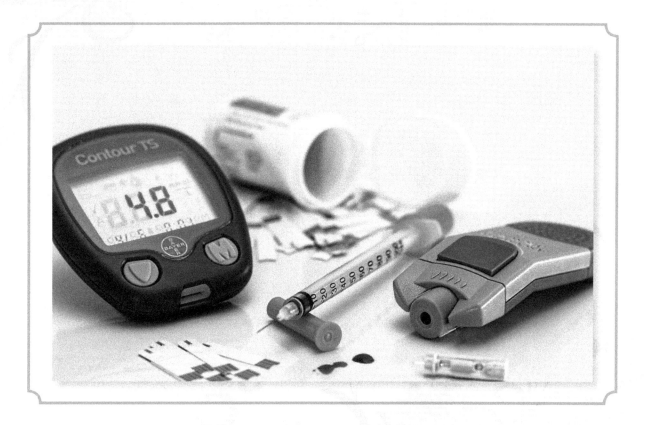

Diabetes has been proposed as a coronary heart disease risk equivalent in an 18-year prospective population-based study in Finnish subjects[Ref 5].

The study concluded that Diabetes without a previous heart attack and a previous heart attack without diabetes indicate a similar risk for coronary heart disease death in men and women. Also, diabetes without any previous evidence of coronary heart disease symptoms, such as heart attack or angina indicates a higher risk than previous evidence of coronary heart disease in non-diabetic subjects, especially in women.

The two diseases are closely associated and can affect each other. High Blood Pressure has the propensity of exacerbating complications of type 2 diabetes. It is most likely that you could develop high blood pressure if you suffer from type 2 diabetes. Also on the flip side of the coin, type 2 diabetes can exacerbate high blood pressure leading to serious cardiovascular problems because diabetes can damage arteries and cause hardening of the arteries. This, in turn, can lead to more serious conditions, such as heart attack, heart failure, stroke, kidney failure or retinopathy leading to blindness if not treated.

In the United Kingdom, about 50% of people aged over 65, and a quarter of all middle-aged adults have high blood pressure. High blood pressure appears to be more common amongst diabetic sufferers. According to a study published in JAMA in September 2015[Ref 6], nearly half of adult population in the US had diabetes or pre-diabetes and based on recent statistics from the American Diabetes Association; nearly 71,000 persons die annually in the US due to complications associated with diabetes. According to a new study published in the Journal of the American Medical Association JAMA[Ref 7], nearly 12% of Chinese adults today (about 113.9 million people) are suffering from diabetes, while less than one percent of the Chinese population was diabetic in 1980. The JAMA study indicates that the common occurrence of the disease has increased along with overweight and obesity as a result of China's economic development.

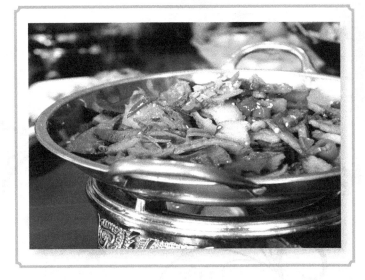

China's diabetes rates have become the highest in the world since the population has become wealthier, adopting the western lifestyle and consuming more animal products.

Diabetes appears to be an alarming epidemic amongst wealthy nations. In fact, type 2 diabetes is a lifestyle disease which is closely associated with obesity, poor diet and sedentary lifestyle. Diet with excessive consumption of meat, fish, eggs, dairy and saturated fats has been found as the major factor for developing type 2 diabetes. China's diabetes rates have become the highest in the world since the population has become wealthier, adopting the western lifestyle and consuming more animal products, including meat, fish, eggs and dairy, while before 1980, the traditional Chinese diet was more bias towards plant-based with little meat or animal product consumption. Also, milk and dairy products were not traditionally a part of the Chinese diet until the influx of western import after the opening up of China to the world.

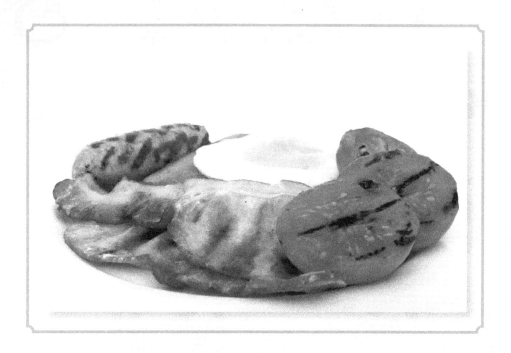

Processed meat, particularly poultry consumption poses a significant risk of developing type 2 diabetes and dementia.

In a recent study, it is found meat and processed meat, particularly poultry consumption poses a significant risk of developing type 2 diabetes and dementia[Ref 8]. Apart from saturated fatty acids, trans fatty acids, cholesterol, heme iron and other meat constituents may cause oxidative stress and tissue inflammation, it is found that a high level of glycotoxins is found in meat, in particular, roasted, fried and boiled meat can cause tissue injury and directly impact the development of dementia and diabetes. The good news is, clinical studies have also shown that adopting a low-fat and plant-based diet may reverse type 2 diabetes by improving insulin sensitivity and reduce blood sugar level and at the same time it helps with weight loss and reduce cholesterol in your circulation network. A significant lifestyle change by consuming a plant-based diet and adopting a daily exercise regime have significant effects in eliminating the root causes of type 2 diabetes and hypertension and in some cases type 2 diabetes is fully eliminated within weeks.

Medication or oral contraceptives and hypertension

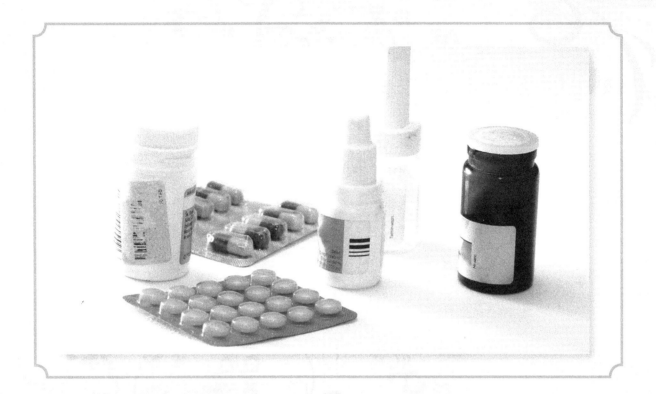

Many medications can cause hypertension symptoms including:

- Many Non-steroidal Anti-inflammatory Drugs (NSAIDs) including both prescription and over-the-counter medication for relieving pain or reducing inflammation from conditions such as arthritis can cause fluid retention and blood pressure to rise.

- Some weight loss drugs or Appetite suppressants can make blood pressure rise and put more stress on your heart. Weight loss drugs are dangerous and unnatural, and should not be taken. If you have an issue with your weight, you should consider eating less and exercising more which is a more effective and healthy way to tackle the problem.

- Some migraine medications work by tightening blood vessels in your head to relieve migraine headaches. By constricting blood vessels throughout your body, these medications can cause your blood pressure rises to a dangerous level.

If you are on any of the above medication, be sure to check it with your physician if you have experienced adverse effects.

Cardiovascular health

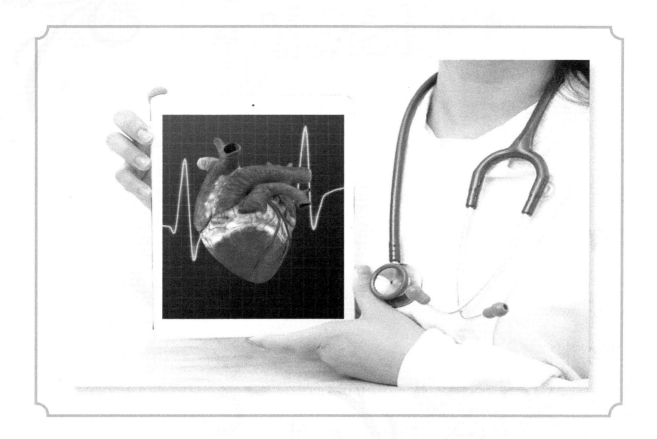

Cardiovascular diseases are the number one cause of death in the world and the leading cause of death in the USA.

The major cause of cardiovascular diseases is atherosclerosis, the hardening, and narrowing of the arteries. The hardening occurs when the walls of the arteries are thickened by fat deposits and calcified plaques, and as a result of the narrowing of the arteries, the body does not get sufficient of blood and oxygen to all the vital organs for the normal body functions. Consequently, the sufferer may experience shortness of breath, tiredness, dizziness, high blood pressure and chest pain. The chest pain is known as angina. Angina is a warning that not only the heart is in distress, it indicates that the atherosclerosis is continuously worsening, leading to blockage of blood supply to the heart and resulting in a heart attack. Likewise, if there is a blockage of the blood supply to the brain, it will trigger a stroke.

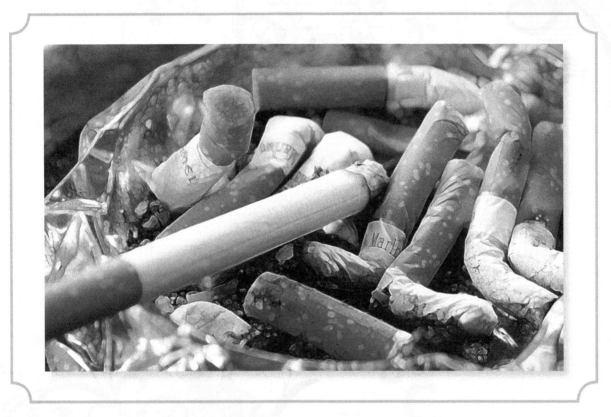

Smoking can cause damage and narrowing of your blood vessels. The risk level rises if you are a long-term heavy smoker or are a woman.

Your smoking can also have a direct impact on the health of your family members via passive smoking from your smoking emission. If you have a family history of cardiovascular disease; you should consider quitting the vice altogether. Your body is a wonderful self-healing mechanism, and it is capable of healing itself once you have quit smoking. Your body can gradually eliminate the toxins and tar from your body when the daily intake of tar and toxic chemicals stops and the oxidation damage and inflammation on the arteries will also gradually subside.

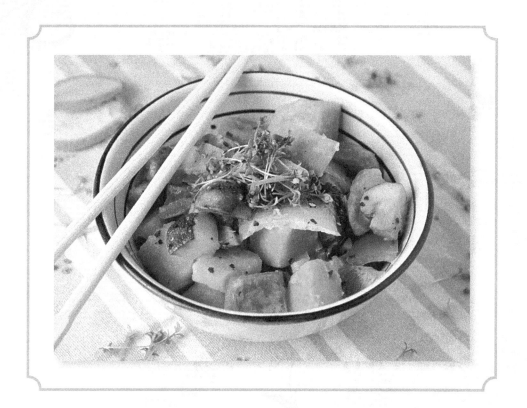

Consider changing to a plant-based diet, a diet with excessive meat and dairy consumption has an adverse consequence to your health.

As we have already discussed in the earlier section **Consider changing to a plant-based diet** on page 36, a diet with excessive meat and dairy consumption has an adverse consequence to your health. Meat and dairy products contain a large quantity of saturated fatty acids, trans fatty acids, cholesterol, heme iron, glycotoxins and other meat constituents that may cause oxidative stress and tissue inflammation leading to plaque formation in your arteries. As a result of hardening and narrowing of your arteries, your blood pressure will elevate as your heart is trying to work harder to pump sufficient blood to supply your body. Changing to a plant-based diet will have a drastic effect of eliminating the plaques and cleaning up your arteries, and when the narrowing reduced, your blood pressure will become normalised again.

High blood pressure is a silent killer when it is undiagnosed or untreated. It is closely related to cardiovascular health. It acts as a double-edged sword when you have developed cardiovascular plaques in your arteries; you are most likely to have high blood pressure, or if you have high blood pressure, your blood vessels are likely to be damaged by the abnormal blood pressure and arterial inflammation. Plaques will be formed as a result of the formation of the lesions causing the thickening of the arterial wall and narrowing of the arteries. Both conditions are echoing each other like a revolving door causing incessant damage to your health and endangering your life. In the worst case scenarios, if plaques rupture, it could lead to a heart attack or a stroke; or your heart could become so enlarged by the excessive workload and the abnormal pressure leading to heart failure.

A sedentary lifestyle and overindulgence of alcohol and food could lead to obesity. Obesity is the root factor of type 2 diabetes, and if you suffer from type 2 diabetes, your cardiovascular health will be compromised as your arteries become hardened by the development of plaques. And as a result of the narrowing of the arteries, your blood pressure elevates to an abnormal level causing further damage to your cardiovascular health. As you can see, all of these conditions are linking to one and other, and they can trigger responses from one and other causing enormous suffering and damage to your health.

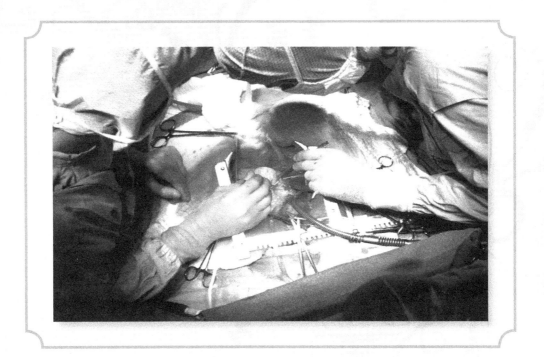

Conquer hypertension and its associated diseases for good

If you have high blood pressure and, or other related conditions as discussed in the previous sections, you should seriously consider taking actions to salvage your health before it is too late because sooner or later they will develop into more life-threatening complications and irreversible conditions:

- Type 2 diabetes can be leading to long-term complications affecting your eyes leading to cataracts, retinopathy, and blindness; damaging your kidneys leading to kidney failure; developing high blood pressure and its complications; damaging nerves leading to peripheral neuropathy, a nerve damage caused by diabetics complications of damage blood vessels; increasing risk of miscarriage and stillbirth with pregnant women and causing erectile dysfunction in men.

- High blood pressure can be leading to cardiovascular diseases, heart attack, aneurysm, heart failure, stroke, dementia, metabolic syndrome and damaging blood vessels in your kidneys.

- Obesity can be leading to type 2 diabetes, high blood pressure and other complications, cardiovascular diseases, gallbladder diseases, cancers, infertility in women and erectile dysfunction in men, osteoarthritis, and fatty liver disease.

Allopathic or conventional medicine is great to alleviate your symptoms or even to save your life when you have an emergency situation caused by these diseases, but it does not eradicate the root causes of these diseases. Indeed, you can choose to take long term medications to maintain a level of physical normality, but it does not equate to a cure. Medications are not nutrition and may be toxic and have adverse side effects of upsetting your natural body synergy and may even cause damage to your body for long-term usage.

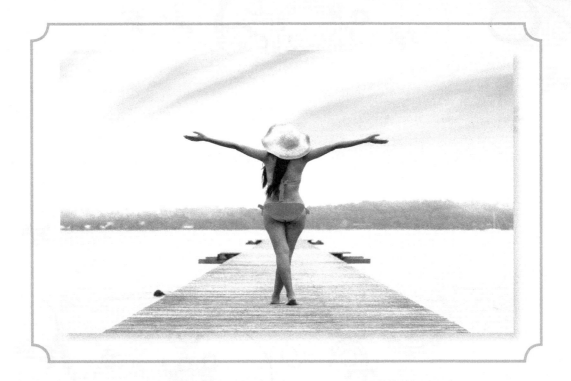

The good news is you can eliminate high blood pressure, cardiovascular diseases, type 2 diabetes, obesity and all other associated conditions naturally if you are determined enough to make a drastic lifestyle change. If you are on long-term medication, consider weaning off your medication slowly, perform acupressure daily and adopt a healthy lifestyle change with the help of a sympathetic physician or a medical professional.

Perform acupressure daily

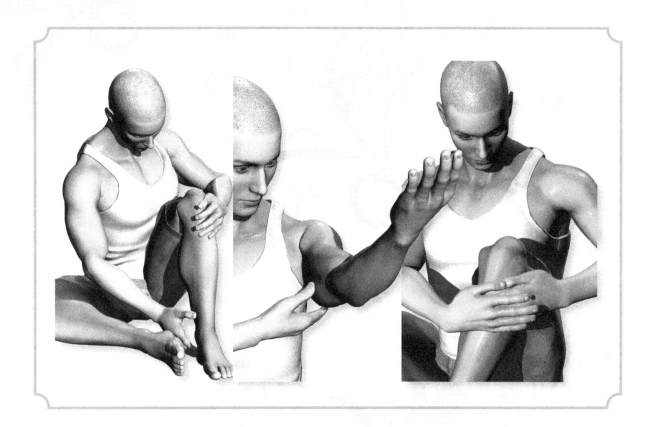

Every journey begins with a single step. Performing acupressure daily to lowering your blood pressure is a positive step to take on your journey of recovery. It is 100% natural and does not require any other medical interventions but most importantly it works instantaneously within 30 minutes. It has a calming effect on your mental well-being by harmonising your Qi (Chi) in your body, and it works synergically with other natural regiments seamlessly such as Qi Gong, Tai Chi, meditation, diet, and exercise.

Examine your diet and learn to eat less and eat wisely

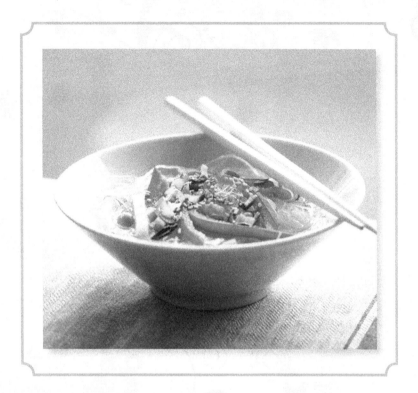

Stop eating when you are 70 to 80% full.

This is a good virtue that has been practised by Taoist monks for many centuries to acquire excellent health and longevity. Eat only when you are hungry. Cut down the portion and chew slowly to appreciate the taste and joy of eating. Stop eating or drinking non-nutritional empty calories junk in between of your meals; that is including soda pop, sweets, chocolates, crisps (chips), biscuits, and ice cream, etc. Stop eating packaged food and you will cut out your refined sugar and trans-fatty acids intake. Refined sugar is an addictive metabolic poison and may cause weight gain, elevated blood sugar and triglycerides, increased uric acid and high blood pressure.

Consider changing to a low-fat plant-based diet. More and more studies and research have provided good scientific evidence that plant-based diet can eliminate cardiovascular diseases, type 2 diabetes, high blood pressure, and even cancers. The double bonus is plant-based diet is also kind to the animals and the environment. It is a common fact that if you are obese and when you have changed to a plant-based diet, your body will shed excessive body weight steadily until it stops at a healthy stable level. Nature has its wonderful way of working miracles, and it is painless because there are no side effects like taking medications.

Use it or lose it

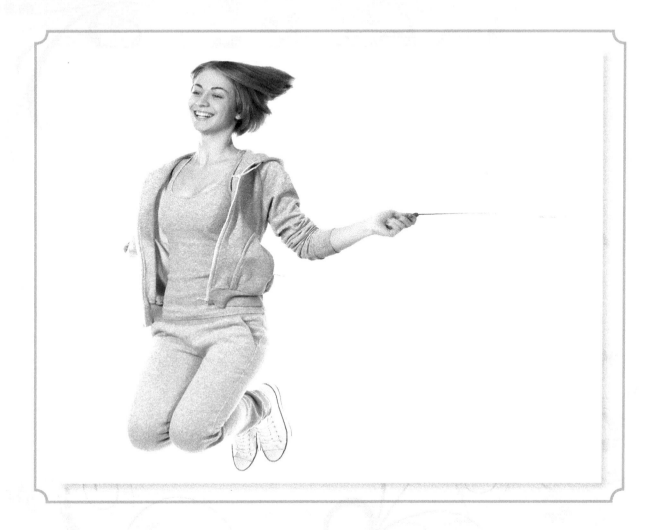

Your body is designed for movements. Exercise controls body weight, boosts production of HDL or and decreases unhealthy triglyceride and keeps your circulation running smoothly, which in turn decreases your risk of developing cardiovascular diseases.

Regular exercise helps nitric oxide production which is a body mechanism for relaxing and dilating the blood vessels to keep your blood pressure normal. When your blood pressure is in good shape, it prevents stroke, metabolic syndrome, type 2 diabetes, cancers, and arthritis. Exercise can reduce stress and dissipates stress hormone adrenaline from your daily fight or flight responses towards, a traffic jam or meeting a difficult client. Most blissfully, Exercise releases happy hormones endorphins and enkephalins which keep your body and mind tranquil, your mood happy and your spirit positive.

Overcome stress

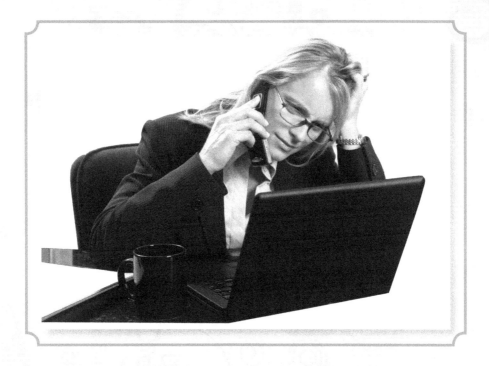

If you are stressed, you should examine your life and find out the root causes which make you worry or unhappy. Remember, stress causes illnesses physically and mentally such as cardiovascular diseases, cancers, depression, ulcer, stroke or physical breakdown. It can elevate your blood pressure to a dangerous level. In Japan, there is even a term called "Karoshi" translated as "overwork death" which occurs amongst the stressful and overworked office clerks. Stress can lead to addiction or take on bad habits such as binging food and alcohol, chain-smoking or even drug abuse when people try to numb their body and mind to cover up the underlining problems and unhappiness.

If you are not happy with your current situation, whether it is a relationship, your job, the place you live or whatever circumstance which is making you unhappy, depressed, or disempowered, consider making a change. Come out of the bad relationship, change your job, look for help medically, psychologically or professionally or do whatever it takes to get yourself out of the situation. Just do something to fix the situation and do not suffer in the silence. Perhaps you need to have a break so that you could re-evaluate your life and to recuperate your body and soul. Don't just work all your life without reaping the fruits of enjoying your life with your family and friends. Learn to be organised so you will save time and avoid the last minute panic and rush. Stop consuming stress induced stimulants, such as caffeine, sugar especially refined sugar such as fructose syrup and white sugar, alcohol or tobacco. Learn to accept life and understand life is not an emergency. Exercise, practise Qi Gong or meditation.

Meditation and prayers

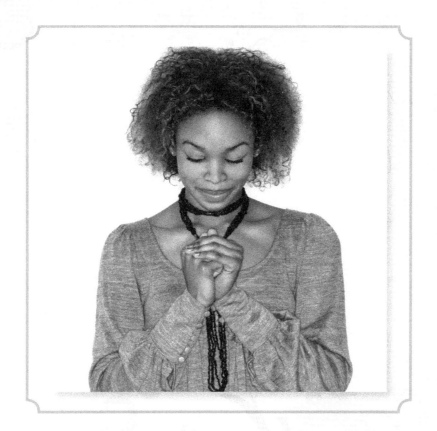

Meditation and prayers are the best ways for one to re-communicate and re-connect with one's higher self or God that you might call it. The internalisation cultivates self-actualisation and promotes a peaceful mind. When your mind is in perfect harmony, your body is also relaxed and have a sense of well-being. When you are calm, you will relinquish your impulse action, anger, impatience and rage, the emotions associated with your fight or flight survival instinct. In such a mindset of calmness and tranquillity, you will affect your surroundings and the people you are associated with. You will emanate love, compassion, and empathy towards others and the people you are dealing with in your everyday life. As your relationships and environments are in harmony and peaceful, you have no cause of stress, anger or unhappiness at all and your body, mind, and spirit will become healthy and in perfect harmony.

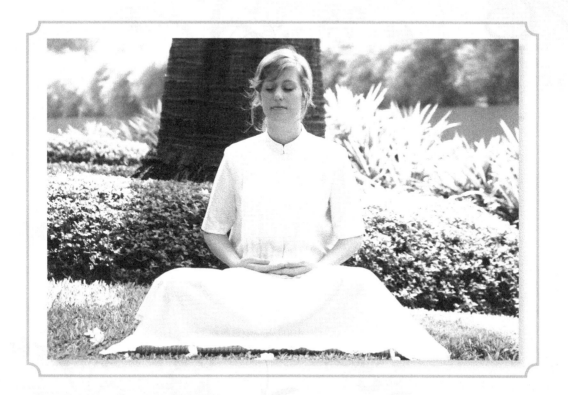

On the contrary, if you are stressed mentally and physically, your body will correspond in a fight or flight mode. The primitive survival instinct takes over and shut off all other major body functions, such as digestion, reproduction or body defence mechanism and immunity. This long-term bombardment of adrenaline saturation and your body's inability to disposing of the hormone will eventually manifest adverse effects affecting your physical, psychological and emotional well-being. As we have already discussed previously, stress can lead to high blood pressure and more serious diseases if you allow your body to shut off your immunity and all major functions for the long term.

Therefore, it is crucial and necessary to give yourself a private moment daily to do your meditation or to communicate with God, your higher self in your prayers. Meditation and prayers can heal your body, mind and soul when you allow yourself to let go totally. Letting go is to release tension, anxiety, anger, sadness, unhappiness and all the negative energy, the major factors that made you ill in the first place. By letting go of all the negative emotions and energy, your body mind and spirit will find peace and harmony within. When you have peace and harmony within, Qi and blood will flow smoothly, and your body will start to heal itself. A harmonised spirit promotes a happy mind and a healthy body.

May all my readers attain happiness,
peace, and harmony in your mind and spirit,
perfect health and vitality to your body.

References

Page 37
Ref1 **Dr T. Colin Campbell**
http://nutritionstudies.org/
Ref2 **Dr T. Colin Campbell China Study**
http://nutritionstudies.org/colin-campbell-china-study-demonstrates-cause-effect/
Ref3 **Dr Dean Ornish's Program for Reversing Heart Disease**
http://deanornish.com/books/
Ref4 **Dr Caldwell Esselstyn's Prevent and Reverse Heart Disease**
http://www.dresselstyn.com/site/books/prevent-reverse/about-the-book/

Page 46
Ref 5 **an 18-year prospective population-based study in Finnish subjects**
http://care.diabetesjournals.org/content/28/12/2901
Ref 6 **According to a study published in JAMA in September 2015**
http://jamanetwork.com/journals/jama/article-abstract/2434682

Page 47
Ref 7 **According to a new study published in the Journal of the American Medical Association JAMA**
http://jamanetwork.com/journals/jama/article-abstract/1812946

Page 48
Ref 8 **In a recent study, it is found meat and processed meat, particularly poultry consumption poses a significant risk of developing type 2 diabetes and dementia.**
http://www.pnas.org/content/111/13/4940

Photograph Acknowledgements

Page 32 Pills *Designed by Bedneyimages - Freepik.com*

Page 36 A bowl of noodles *Designed by Valeria_aksakova - Freepik.com*

Page 37 Skipping *Designed by Yanalya / Freepik.com*

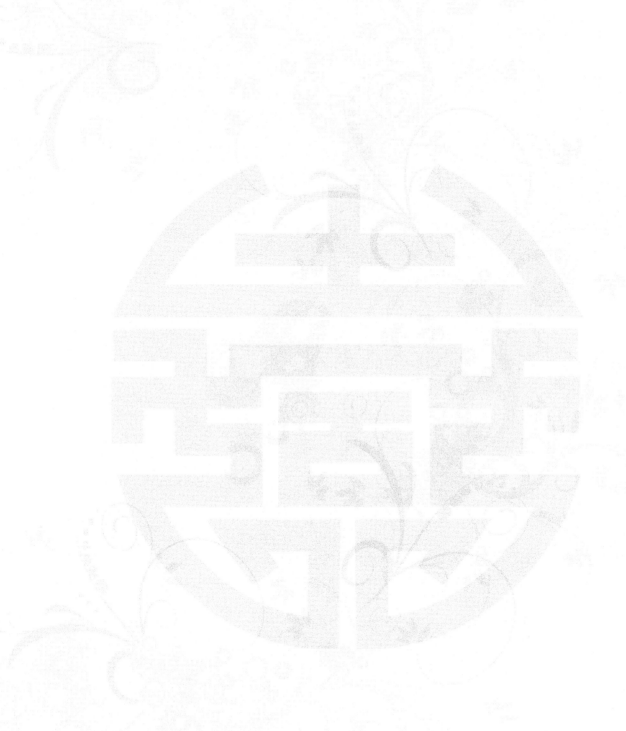

About the author

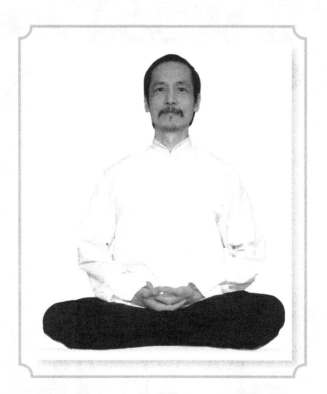

Master Charles Chan has been teaching Taoist healing arts, meditation, Tai Chi, Qi Gong and Shaolin Kung Fu since 1973. He was one of the earliest executive members and technical advisors of the British Kung Fu Council (Now known as the British Council of Chinese Martial Arts) in the 70s and is the founder and chairman of the UK Shaolin Mo Jia Kung Fu Association.

Other Publications

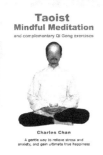

Taoist Mindful Meditation and complementary Qi Gong exercises
A gentle way to relieve stress and anxiety, and gain ultimate true happiness

- Kindle 2nd Edition March 2019
  Published by Taoway Publishing
  ASIN: B07PPT1LHZ

- Paperback (8." x 10") 1st Edition April 2019
  Published by Taoway Publishing
  ISBN 978-0-9957419-6-6

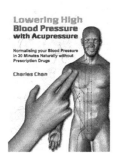

Lowering High Blood Pressure with Acupressure
Normalising your blood pressure in 30 minutes naturally without prescription drugs

- Kindle 2nd Edition February 2017
  Published by Taoway Publishing
  ASIN: B01N0LN0IJ

- Apple iBook 1st Edition April 2017
  Published by Taoway Publishing
  ISBN 978-0-9957419-2-8

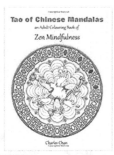

Tao of Chinese Mandalas
An Adult Colouring Book of Zen Mindfulness

- Paperback (8.5" x 11") 1st Edition April 2017
  Published by Taoway Publishing
  ISBN 978-0-9957419-1-1

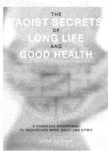

The Taoist Secrets of Long Life and Good Health
A Complete Programme to Rejuvenate Mind, Body and Spirit

- Published by Godsfield Press, a division of the Octopus Publishing Group
  Paper back (10.2" x 7.7") 1st Edition January 2006
  ISBN 1-84181-281-1

For the latest news and other publications, please visit www.taoway.co.uk.

CPSIA information can be obtained
at www.ICGtesting.com
Printed in the USA
LVHW071547170920
666362LV00016B/1568